I0410495

Health Adviser: Hypertension

Bennett Obi

ISBN -10 :153902539X
ISBN-13: 978- 1539025399

CONTENTS

Chapter One

Hypertension and Risk Factors

What is Hypertension? Hypertension also known as High Blood Pressure is a sustained increase in blood pressure reading above the normal.

Overview:

As of 2014, approximately one billion adults or ~22% of the population of the world have hypertension. It is estimated that 50 million or more Americans have high BP warranting some form of treatment. It is also estimated that globally approximately 7.1 million deaths per year may be attributable to hypertension.

It is slightly more frequent in men, in those of low socioeconomic status and prevalence increases with age. It is common in high, medium and low income countries. The prevalence of raised blood pressure is highest in Africa, (30% for both sexes) and lowest in the WHO Region of the Americas (18% for both sexes). Rates also vary markedly within WHO regions with rates as low as 3.4% (men) and 6.8% (women) in rural India and as high as 68.9% (men) and 72.5% (women) in Poland. In Europe hypertension occurs in about 30-45% of people as of 2013. In 1995 it was estimated that 43 million people (24% of the populations) in the United States had hypertension or were taking antihypertensive medication. By 2004 this had increased to 29% and further to 34% (76 million US adults) by 2006. African American adults in the United States have among the highest rates of hypertension in the world at 44%. It is also more common in Filipino Americans and less common in US whites and Mexican Americans.

But before we go further let us try to understand what blood pressure is. **Blood pressure (BP)** is the pressure exerted by circulating blood upon the walls of blood vessels. Blood pressure is usually expressed in terms of the systolic (maximum) pressure over diastolic (minimum) pressure and is measured in millimeters of mercury (mm Hg).

BP $\frac{\text{systolic}}{\text{diastolic}}$ **(read systolic over diastolic)**

The systolic pressure is the maximum pressure exerted on the blood vessel walls when the heart contracts to pump out blood. The diastolic pressure is the minimum pressure on the blood vessel walls when the heart relaxes to refill again (pressure at rest).

It is measured using an instrument called sphygmomanometer. This sphygmomanometer has the mercury type and the aneroid type. The aneroid type has manual and digital forms. The digital form is convenient to use but the readings are less reliable. The user has to take two or more readings and find the average. The aneroid sphygmomanometer also has the arm and wrist types. For self-monitoring of blood pressure either of them is okay, it all depends on choice.

It is important to observe these simple rules below when measuring the blood pressure.

- Don't drink coffee or smoke cigarettes for 30 minutes prior to the test.

- Go to the bathroom before the test.

- Sit for 5 minutes before the test.

Risk Factors for hypertension (factors that make someone more prone to the development of hypertension than others):

Anyone can develop high blood pressure; however, age, race or ethnicity, being overweight, gender, lifestyle habits, and a family history of high blood pressure can increase the risk for developing high blood pressure.

Age

Blood pressure tends to rise with age. In America, for instance about 65 percent of people aged 60 years or older have high blood pressure.

Race/Ethnicity

High blood pressure is more common in African American adults than in Caucasian or Hispanic American adults. The African Americans also tend to get high blood pressure earlier in life.

Overweight

Overweight or obese people are more likely to develop prehypertension or high blood pressure.

Gender

Before age 55, men are more likely than women to develop high blood pressure. After age 55, women are more likely than men to develop high blood pressure.

Lifestyle Habits

Unhealthy lifestyle habits can raise the risk for high blood pressure, and they include:

- Eating too much sodium or too little potassium

- Lack of physical activity

- Drinking too much alcohol

- Stress

Family History

A family history of high blood pressure raises the risk of developing prehypertension or high blood pressure. Some people have a high sensitivity to sodium and salt, which may increase their risk for high blood pressure and may run in families. Genetic causes of this condition are why family history is a risk factor for this condition.

An individual's blood pressure varies with exercise, emotional reactions, sleep, digestion and time of day. The blood pressure is lowest during sleep. The blood pressure tends to be at its best early in the morning when the individual is free from stress and emotional disturbances.

Blood Circulation and the heart

When the heart contracts, the contraction generates the force that drives blood through the circulatory system in a cycle that delivers oxygen, nutrients and chemicals to the body's cells and removes cellular waste. When it relaxes, it receives the blood from the tissues and all the waste products that it collects while circulating through the body. This blood returns to the heart through the venous system. The quantity of blood returning to the heart effectively determines the quantity of blood the heart pumps out – its cardiac output. This is because the heart effectively pumps out all the blood that it receives.

Blood pressure is directly proportional to the amount of blood that flows through the vascular system in one minute **(called cardiac output CO)** and the resistance that the blood encounters while flowing through the blood vessels **(called peripheral resistance PR).** If the cardiac output increases, while the PR remains the same, the BP will increase. If the PR increases while the cardiac output remains the same, the blood pressure will rise. If both the cardiac output and the peripheral resistance increase, the blood pressure will increase more. So anything that affects the cardiac output and/or peripheral resistance will affect the blood pressure.

Blood pressure is regulated by **the nervous system and endocrine system**.

The **sympathetic nervous system,** when it is activated tends to push the blood pressure up, while the **parasympathetic nervous system** tends to lower it.

Excess **adrenal gland hormones and thyroid hormones** tend to push up the blood pressure. The absence of these hormones tend to lower the blood pressure.

The action of the hormones on the blood vessels affects the **muscle tone and the elasticity** of the blood vessels making the vessels to either **constrict** (become narrower) or **dilate** (expand to become wider).

When the vessels constrict, the resistance to blood flow increases and when the vessels dilate the resistance to blood flow in the vessels is decreased.

Since the blood pressure increases with increase in the peripheral resistance, any condition that increases the peripheral resistance, increases the blood pressure.

The converse is also true; any condition that lowers the peripheral resistance lowers the blood pressure.

It is not only the effect of hormones on the blood vessels that can narrow the blood vessels.

Mechanical blocking like the deposition of fatty plaques along the inner surface of the vessels can make the vessels narrow thereby increasing the peripheral resistance and ultimately the blood pressure.

Some congenital malformations or disease-induced malformations, trauma-induced malformations can narrow the blood vessels, thus increasing the resistance to blood flow and ultimately increasing the blood pressure.

The **viscosity** of blood also affects the speed with which the blood flows through the arteries. Thick blood (haemoconcentrated blood) moves slowly through the blood vessels and makes more contact with the vessel walls, while dilute blood flows faster through the blood vessels with less contact with the vessel walls. Making contact with the blood vessel walls increases the peripheral resistance.

Any condition that increases the volume of blood in circulation will increase the cardiac output. Since increase in the cardiac output will result in the increase in blood pressure, it follows that any increase in the blood volume will lead to increase in the blood pressure.

The converse is also true; any condition that reduces the blood volume e g haemorrhage (rapid blood loss), diarrhoea and vomiting will reduce the blood pressure.

Low blood pressure (also called hypotension) results only in disease conditions and is always associated with symptoms. Any low blood pressure that is not associated with symptoms is normal blood pressure for that individual even when it is lower than the generally accepted normal blood pressure.

The table below shows the classification of the blood pressure in the adult human being. The normal blood pressure is a range of values and not a specific value.

Classification of blood pressure:

Classification of blood pressure for adults (JNC7)[1]

Category	systolic, mm Hg	diastolic, mm Hg
Normal	90–119	60–79
High normal (Prehypertension)	120–139	80–89
Stage 1 hypertension	140–159	90–99
Stage 2 hypertension	160–179	100–109
Stage 3 hypertension (Hypertensive	≥180	≥110

---

[1] Seventh report of the Joint National Committee on Prevention, Detection, Evaluation and treatment of HBP.

emergency)		
Isolated systolic hypertension	≥140	<90

Hypertension also known as high blood pressure is defined as sustained increase in the blood pressure above the normal range. An isolated increase in either the systolic or the diastolic blood pressure recording should be disregarded but the individual should be under observation. A persistent high systolic value even when the diastolic value is normal is called systolic hypertension. It should be treated. A persistent diastolic reading even when the systolic reading is normal, is called diastolic hypertension. It should be treated.

Prehypertension is **not** a disease category. But individuals with prehypertension are at high risk of developing hypertension. Such individuals should practice lifestyle modifications to prevent or at least delay the development of hypertension. However if individuals with prehypertension have diabetes or kidney disease in addition, they should be considered for treatment if lifestyle modification fails to reduce their BP to 130/80 or less.

All people with hypertension (stages 1 and 2) should be treated.

Cardiovascular Disease Risk

The risk of cardiovascular disease is directly related to the severity of hypertension whether the individual has other risk factors or not. The higher the BP, the greater the chance of heart attack, heart failure (HF), stroke, and kidney diseases. The presence of each additional risk factor will only worsen the risk from hypertension. The risk factors should be managed according to available guidelines to minimize the risk of cardiovascular disease.

Systolic blood pressure (SBP) and Cardiovascular diseases (CVDs)

Studies have shown that SBP is a major risk factor for CVDs. The rise in SBP continues throughout life in contrast to diastolic blood pressure (DBP), which rises until approximately age 50, tends to level off over the next decade, and may remain the same or fall later in life. Diastolic hypertension predominates before age 50, either alone or in combination with SBP elevation.

The prevalence of systolic hypertension increases with age, and above 50 years of age, systolic hypertension represents the most common form of hypertension. DBP is a more potent cardiovascular risk factor than SBP until age 50; thereafter, SBP is more important.

Controlling isolated systolic hypertension reduces total mortality, cardiovascular mortality, stroke, and HF events.

Types of Hypertension

1. Primary Hypertension

Most hypertension (90-95%) do not have any identifiable cause. Such hypertension are called primary hypertension or essential hypertension. They are due to nonspecific lifestyle and genetic factors. Lifestyle factors that increase the risk include:

- Excessive consumption of salt (sodium chloride), in excess of 6 grams daily (normal salt intake is 3-6 grams daily)
- Obesity (excess body weight)
- Smoking
- Excessive alcohol consumption.
- Lack of physical activity
- Stress

- Older age (hypertension is more common in old age due to changes in the blood vessels. The blood vessels become stiff and some are partially blocked by atherosclerosis (plaques deposits))
- Diabetes Mellitus
- Insufficient intake of potassium, calcium, and magnesium;

2. Secondary Hypertension:

Secondary hypertension is that type of hypertension that has an identifiable cause; they constitute 5-10 % of all hypertension cases.

They are due to an identifiable cause, such as;

- Chronic kidney diseases
- Renal artery disease (narrowing of the kidney arteries)
- Endocrine disorders like, thyroid and adrenal gland disorders -- hyperthyroidism, hyperaldosteronism, Cushing's disease etc.
- The use of birth control pills.

- Family history of hypertension
- Genetics
- Sleep apnoea (a condition characterized by pauses in breathing or periods of shallow breathing during sleep)

Children and Hypertension

It is true that hypertension is a disease of old people but hypertension also affects children and adolescents even infants and neonates. In young infants and neonates, hypertension is associated failure to thrive, seizures, irritability, lack of energy, and difficulty with breathing. In older infants and children, hypertension can cause headache, unexplained irritability, fatigue, failure to thrive, blurred vision, nosebleeds, and facial paralysis.

Rates of high blood pressure in children and adolescents have increased in the last 20 years in the United States. Childhood hypertension, particularly in pre-adolescents, is more often secondary to an underlying disorder than in adults. Kidney disease is the most common secondary cause of hypertension in children and adolescents. Nevertheless, primary or essential hypertension accounts for most cases.

Chapter Two

Symptoms of Hypertension

Hypertension is essentially a symptomless condition (meaning that it does not have symptoms). Many people do not talk about the symptoms of high blood pressure, they prefer to refer to it as the myth of the symptoms and Signs of high blood pressure. According to the America Heart Association "There's a common misconception that people with high blood pressure, also called HBP or hypertension, will experience symptoms such as nervousness, sweating, difficulty sleeping or facial flushing. The truth is that HBP is largely a symptomless condition. If people ignore their blood pressure because they think symptoms will alert them to the problem, they are taking a dangerous chance with their life. Everybody needs to know their blood pressure numbers, and everyone needs to prevent high blood pressure from developing"[2].

The myth of symptomatic headaches

The best evidence indicates that high blood pressure does not cause headaches except perhaps in the case of hypertensive crisis (systolic/top number higher than 180 OR diastolic/bottom number higher than 110)[3].

In the early 1900s, it was assumed that headaches were more common among people with high blood pressure. However, research into the subject doesn't support this view. According to one study, people with high blood pressure seem to have significantly fewer headaches than the general population.

In a study published in the journal *Neurology*, people with higher systolic blood pressure (the

---

2

www.heart.org/.../HighBloodPressure/SymptomsDiagnosisMonitoringofHighBloodPressure March 23, 2016.

3

www.heart.org/.../HighBloodPressure/SymptomsDiagnosisMonitoringofHighBloodPressure March 23, 2016.

top number in blood pressure readings) were up to 40 percent *less* likely to have headaches compared to those with healthier blood pressure readings.

Therefore, headaches or the lack of headaches are not reliable indicators of your blood pressure. Instead, work with your doctor and know your numbers[4].

The myth of symptomatic nosebleeds

Except with hypertensive crisis, nosebleeds are not a reliable indicator for HBP. In one study, 17 percent of people treated for high blood pressure emergencies at the hospital had nosebleeds. However, 83 percent reported no such symptom. Although it's also been noted that some people in the early stages of high blood pressure may have more nosebleeds than usual, there are other possible explanations. If your nosebleeds are frequent (more than once a week) or if they are

---

[4]www.heart.org/.../HighBloodPressure/SymptomsDiagnosisMonitoringofHighBloodPressure March 23, 2016

heavy or hard to stop, you should talk to your healthcare professional.

Keep in mind that nosebleeds can be caused by a variety of factors, with the most common one being dry air. The lining of the nose contains many tiny blood vessels that can bleed easily. In a hot climate like the desert Southwest or with heated indoor air, the nasal membranes can dry out and make the nose more susceptible to bleeding. Other causes include vigorously blowing your nose; medical conditions like allergies, colds, sinusitis or a deviated septum; and side effects from some anticoagulant drugs like warfarin (Coumadin®) or aspirin[5].

Even though some people with high blood pressure report symptoms like headaches (particularly at the back of the head and in the morning), as well as lightheadedness, vertigo (dizziness), tinnitus (buzzing or hissing in the

---

[5]

www.heart.org/.../HighBloodPressure/SymptomsDiagnosisMonitoringofHighBloodPressure March 23, 2016 ears), altered vision or fainting episodes. These symptoms, however, might be related to associated anxiety rather than the high blood pressure itself.

Chapter Three

Complications of Hypertension

High blood pressure affects every organ in the body adversely. High blood pressure (hypertension) can quietly damage the human body for years before symptoms develop. If left uncontrolled, the sufferer could end up with a disability, a poor quality of life or even a fatal heart attack. Fortunately, with treatment and lifestyle changes, high blood pressure could be controlled and the risk of life-threatening complications reduced.

When high blood pressure is not effectively controlled, a lot of complications could result.

1. Damage to the arteries

Arteries are blood vessels that carry oxygen-rich blood from the heart to other parts of the body including the heart itself.

Healthy arteries are flexible, strong and elastic. Their inner lining is smooth so that blood flows freely, supplying vital organs and tissues with adequate nutrients and oxygen. But with hypertension, the increased pressure of blood flowing through the arteries gradually damages the blood vessels making them less elastic, narrower and rigid.

High blood pressure can damage the endothelium (the cells lining the inner surface of the arteries). The damage to the endothelium initiates a process of events that make artery walls thick and stiff. That disease is called arteriosclerosis or hardening of the arteries. When fats from the diet enter the bloodstream, the damaged cells could trap them and fat molecules then collect to start atherosclerosis. (Atherosclerosis is a disease in which plaque builds up inside the arteries).

Plaque is made up of fat, cholesterol, calcium, and other substances found in the blood. Over the time, plaque hardens and narrows the arteries. This narrowing of the arteries impedes the flow of oxygen-rich blood to the organs and other parts of the body.

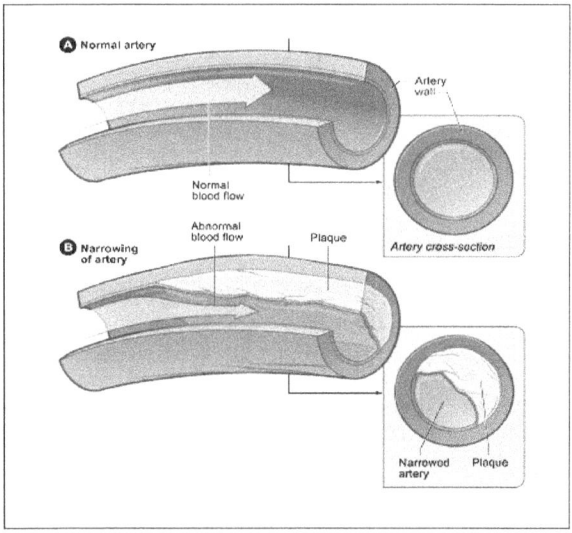

Figure 1 Atherosclerosis

Figure A shows a normal artery with normal blood flow. The inset image shows a cross-section of a normal artery. Figure B shows an artery with plaque build-up. The inset image shows a cross-section of an artery with plaque build-up.

These changes, that is, the arteriosclerosis and atherosclerosis, can affect arteries throughout the body, thereby impeding blood flow to the heart, kidneys, brain, arms and legs. The damage can cause many problems, including chest pain (angina), heart attack, heart failure, kidney failure, stroke, blocked arteries in the legs or arms (peripheral artery disease), eye damage, and aneurysms. It could be rightly said that the single most important cause of complication by hypertension is the damage to the arteries.

Aneurysm: As the high blood pressure continues uncontrolled, with time, the constant pressure of blood moving through a weakened artery could cause a section of its wall to enlarge and form a bulge. That bulge is called aneurysm. As time goes on, if the high blood pressure is not controlled, the aneurysm continues to enlarge and could eventually rupture. If it ruptures, it could cause life-threatening internal bleeding. Aneurysms can form in any artery throughout the body, but they are most common in the aorta, the largest artery in the human body.

2. Complications affecting the brain:

i. Stroke: Uncontrolled hypertension could cause stroke. Stroke is when poor blood flow to the brain results in cell death. There are two main types of stroke: ischemic stroke due to lack of blood flow, and hemorrhagic, due to bleeding. Stroke results when the damaged blood vessel supplying some part of the brain ruptures (bursts), causing bleeding in the brain (haemorrhagic stroke). The blood supply to that part of the brain is cut off and the brain tissues eventually die. The part of the body that is served by that part of the brain will cease to function. If the bleeding is in the left part of the brain, the effect will be felt on the right part of the body. If the bleeding occurs in the right side of the brain, the left part of the body will be affected. This is because the right part of the brain (right cerebral hemisphere) controls the functions of the left part of the body. While the left part of the brain (left cerebral hemisphere) controls the

functions of the right part of the body.
The accumulation of blood inside the skull,
which is a bony structure, does not allow room
for expansion so the bleeding causes a lot of
pressure on the brain substance thereby causing
more damage to the brain tissues. So
haemorrhagic stroke causes stroke not only by
cutting off the blood supply to a part of the brain
but also by exerting pressure to the brain tissues.
Ischemic stroke results when the blood vessel
supplying a part of the brain is blocked by either
the deposits on the inner surface of the blood
vessel or by a blood clot flowing in the blood
stream. The resultant effect is death of cells distal
to the point of blockage (occlusion). This effect
results because the brain, like the heart has end
arteries, meaning that the arteries of the brain do
not form anastomosis. In so many parts of the
body, the blood vessels form anastomosis so that
when an artery is blocked, the surrounding

arteries will take over the functions of the blocked vessel through the anastomosis.

The incidence of stroke rises progressively with increasing blood pressure levels, particularly systolic blood pressure in individuals >65 years. Fortunately convincingly controlling the blood pressure decreases the incidence of both ischemic and hemorrhagic strokes.

ii. **Transient ischemic attack** (TIA). Sometimes called a ministroke, a transient ischemic attack is a brief, temporary disruption of blood supply to the brain. It is often caused by atherosclerosis or a blood clot — both of which can arise from high blood pressure. **A transient ischemic attack is often a warning that the individual is at risk of a full-blown stroke.**

A person with TIA may experience some of the following symptoms:

Face – the face may have dropped on one side, the person may not be able to smile, or their mouth or eye may have dropped.

Arms –the person may not be able to lift both arms due to weakness or numbness.

Speech– the speech may be slurred or garbled, or the person may not be able to talk at all, despite appearing to be awake.

Paralysis – there could be complete paralysis of one side of the body

Vision – there could be sudden loss or blurring of vision

Dizziness – the person may experience a spell of dizziness

Confusion – there could be a brief episode of confusion, or difficulty understanding what others are saying

Balance – there could be problems with balance and co-ordination

Dysphagia – there could be difficulty with swallowing (dysphagia)

The symptoms of TIA usually disappears after a short time, though some may last longer. The person usually recovers completely but should seek medical advice.

iii. **Dementia**. Dementia is a brain disease resulting in problems with thinking, speaking, reasoning, memory, vision and movement. It results from inadequate blood supply to the brain, which is caused by the effect of uncontrolled high blood pressure on the arteries. It could result from other conditions that could lead to the narrowing and blockage of the arteries that supply blood to the brain.

iv. **Mild cognitive impairment (MCI).** It means a mild form of impairment of cognition. (Cognition is the mental action or process of acquiring knowledge and understanding through thought, experience, and the senses. It encompasses processes such as knowledge, attention, memory and working memory, judgment and evaluation, reasoning and "computation", problem solving and decision making, comprehension and production of language, etc. Human cognition is conscious and unconscious, concrete or abstract, as well as intuitive (like knowledge of a language) and conceptual (like a model of a language). Cognitive processes use existing knowledge and generate new knowledge).

So when someone has mild cognitive impairment, it means that the person is gradually losing that power of mental action or process of acquiring knowledge and understanding. Mild cognitive impairment is a transition stage between the changes in understanding and memory that come with aging and the more-serious problems caused by Alzheimer's disease. Like dementia, it can result from blocked blood flow to the brain when high blood pressure damages arteries.

Mild cognitive impairment causes cognitive changes that are serious enough to be noticed by the individuals experiencing them or to other people, but the changes are not severe enough to interfere with daily life or independent function. Those with MCI have an increased risk of eventually developing Alzheimer's or another type of dementia. However, not all people with MCI get worse and some eventually get better.

Long-term studies suggest that 10 to 20 percent of those aged 65 years and older may have MCI. Experts classify Mild cognitive impairment based on the thinking skills affected:

MCI that primarily affects memory is known as "amnestic MCI." With amnestic MCI, a person may start to forget important information that they would previously have recalled easily, such as appointments, conversations or recent events.

MCI that affects thinking skills other than memory is known as "non-amnestic MCI." Thinking skills that may be affected by non-amnestic MCI include the ability to make sound decisions, judge the time or sequence of steps needed to complete a complex task, or visual perception.

v. Hypertensive encephalopathy: It is a very serious condition caused by uncontrolled hypertension. It is characterized by headache, nausea and vomiting, alterations in mental status and focal neurological signs. If hypertensive encephalopathy is left untreated, it could run a progressive course through stupor, coma, seizures (convulsions) and death in a matter of hours.

3. **Complications affecting the eyes (hypertensive retinopathy):** Through the same process of damaging the blood vessels, uncontrolled hypertension could initiate many changes in the eyes leading eventually to blindness.

4. Complications affecting the kidneys: (hypertensive nephropathy)

In the same way hypertension damages blood vessels supplying the organs of the body, so it damages blood vessels to the kidneys. The compromised blood supply to the kidneys gradually damages the functional units (nephrons) of the kidney thereby causing injury and end stage renal diseases (ESRD). ESRD is the irreversible stage of kidney damage. It can only be treated by dialysis or kidney transplant.

The risk to the kidneys appears to be more closely related to systolic than the diastolic blood pressure. This means that people with systolic hypertension are more likely to have early kidney damages.

The black men are at greater risk than white men for developing ESRD at every level of blood pressure.

The appearance of protein (albumin) and creatinine in tested urine sample is an early indication of kidney damage. It is also a risk factor for renal disease progression and for cardiovascular disease.

5. Complications affecting the heart

(Left ventricular hypertrophy, Hypertensive cardiomyopathy, and Myocardial infarction)

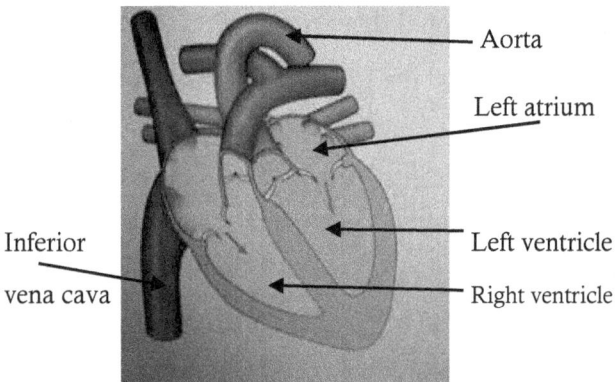

Figure 2: Cross section of the human heart

The heart diseases caused by hypertension are due to both structural and functional adaptations. When the left ventricle, which is the part of the heart that pumps blood from the heart to the other parts of the body, has to work extra hard to pump blood through the damaged and narrowed blood vessels, its muscles become thicker and stiff. That situation is called **left ventricular hypertrophy**.

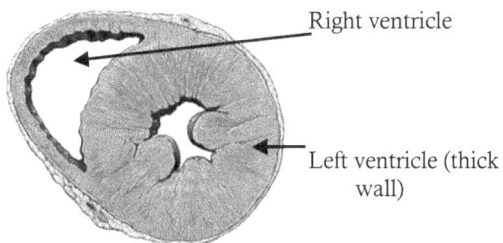

Right ventricle

Left ventricle (thick wall)

Figure 3: Left ventricular hypertrophy

The heart becomes larger because the left ventricle has become thicker and larger. This left ventricular hypertrophy leads to another condition called **diastolic dysfunction**. Diastolic dysfunction is a situation in which the left ventricle is not able to relax very well during diastole to receive all the blood from the body. That condition leads to **heart failure**.

Heart failure (HF), often referred to as congestive heart failure (CHF), occurs when the heart is unable to pump enough blood to meet the body's needs. A person with heart failure usually shows signs and symptoms like **shortness of breath, excessive tiredness, and leg swelling.** The shortness of breath is usually worse with exercise or while lying down. It could wake the person up at night with strong coughing. The person also has a limited ability to exercise.

People with left ventricular hypertrophy are at increased risk for stroke, CHF, and sudden death.

The damage to the arteries supplying the heart (coronary arteries) could lead to death of some part of the heart muscle. This condition is called **myocardial infarction or heart attack.**

Uncontrolled hypertension could also cause **irregularity of heart beats** (arrhythmias).

Fortunately aggressive control of hypertension can regress or reverse left ventricular hypertrophy and reduce the risk of cardiovascular disease.

Left ventricular hypertrophy is seen in 25% of the hypertensive patients and can easily be diagnosed by using echocardiography.

6. Sexual dysfunction

The narrowing and hardening of the blood vessels caused by hypertension limits blood flow to the penis and makes it difficult for men to achieve and maintain erection.

Women also have limited blood flow to their vagina due to the same reasons. For some women, this leads to a decrease in sexual desire or arousal, vaginal dryness, or difficulty achieving orgasm. This sexual dysfunction causes anxiety and relationship issues for both men and women.

7. Complications associated to diabetes and hypertension

Diabetes has several complications, one of which is hypertension or high blood pressure. Data indicate that at least 60-80 percent of individuals who develop diabetes will eventually develop high blood pressure. The high blood pressure is gradual at early stages and may take at least 10–15 years to fully develop.

Apart from diabetes, other factors that might cause high blood pressure are obesity, insulin resistance and high cholesterol levels.

Generally it has been observed that many people with diabetes have poor control of blood pressure. Less than 25 percent of diabetics have good control of their blood pressure. The presence of high blood pressure in diabetes is associated with a fourfold increase in death chiefly from heart disease and strokes.

The chief reason why people with diabetes develop high blood pressure is hardening of the arteries. Diabetes tends to speed up the process of atherosclerosis.

The other fact about diabetes is that it affects both large and small blood vessels in the body. Over time, blood vessels become clogged with fatty depots, become non-compliant and lose their elasticity. The process of atherosclerosis is a lot faster in diabetic individuals who do not have good control of their blood sugars.

The high blood pressure eventually leads to heart failure, strokes, heart attacks, blindness, kidney failure, loss of libido and poor circulation of blood in the legs. When the blood supply to the feet is compromised, the chances of infections and amputations also increase.

All diabetics should know that even mild elevations in blood pressure can be detrimental to health. Studies have shown that diabetics with even a slight elevation in blood pressure have 2-3 times the risk of heart disease compared to individuals without diabetes.

Other possible dangers of high blood pressure

High blood pressure can also affect other areas of the body, leading to such problems as:

- **Bone loss.** High blood pressure can increase loss of calcium in the urine. That excessive elimination of calcium may lead to loss of bone density (osteoporosis), which in turn can lead to fractures (pathological fractures), meaning that bones just break without trauma. The risk is especially increased in older women (post menopause).

- **Trouble with sleeping.** Many people with hypertension have obstructive sleep apnoea — a condition in which the throat muscles relax causing the person to snore loudly. Sleep apnoea occurs in more than half of the people with high blood pressure. It's now thought that high blood pressure itself may help trigger sleep apnoea. Also, sleep deprivation resulting from sleep apnoea can raise the blood pressure.

Hypertensive emergencies

Although high blood pressure is typically a chronic condition that gradually causes damage over the years, in some cases the blood pressure could rise very quickly and severely (above 180/110) that it becomes a medical emergency requiring immediate treatment, often with hospitalization.

Consequences of hypertensive emergency on the brain include **memory loss, personality changes, trouble concentrating, irritability or progressive loss of consciousness (encephalopathy).**

In these situations, high blood pressure can cause **stroke.**

It could cause severe **damage to the body's main artery (aortic dissection).**

In pregnancy it leads to **seizures (preeclampsia or eclampsia).**

Hypertensive emergencies could cause **unstable chest pain** (angina) and **heart attack.**

It could cause **sudden impaired pumping of the heart,** leading to fluid backup in the lungs resulting in shortness of breath (pulmonary oedema).

It could lead to **sudden loss of kidney function** (acute renal failure).

It could lead to rupture of retinal artery leading to **bleeding inside the eye, blurring of vision or even blindness.**

In most cases, these emergencies arise because high blood pressure hasn't been adequately controlled.

When hypertensive emergency occurs in pregnancy, it is a disaster. It usually occurs in the second half of pregnancy and following delivery. It is usually diagnosed by elevated blood pressure, protein in the urine and swelling of the legs usually detected during a routine check because it has no symptoms.

Hypertension occurs in 8- 10% of pregnancies, and 5% of those gestational hypertension will progress to preeclampsia, which is a very serious condition.

Elevated blood pressure (140/90) without protein in urine is called **gestational hypertension or pregnancy-induced hypertension**. Elevated blood pressure in pregnancy that is associated with leg swelling and protein in urine is called **preeclampsia**. Preeclampsia with symptoms like headache, epigastric pain, seizures, visual disturbances, vomiting and marked leg swelling, is **eclampsia.**

Preeclampsia is a very serious condition accounting for approximately 16% of all maternal deaths globally. It also doubles the risk of perinatal mortality. When a pregnant woman with preeclampsia starts showing symptoms like headache, visual disturbances (seeing halos), vomiting, epigastric pain (pain over the stomach) then the more serious condition called eclampsia is imminent. The woman must be hospitalized and managed aggressively, if not death will follow.

Eclampsia is the real hypertensive emergency that has several serious complications including vision loss, brain swelling, seizures, kidney failure, pulmonary edema, and disseminated intravascular coagulation (DIC). DIC is a blood-clotting disorder in which the blood fails to clot and the woman can die of excessive blood loss.

Chapter Four

Management of Hypertension

Management of hypertension involves

- **Prevention,**

- **Treatment plan and**

- **Medicines.**

1. **Prevention**: People who are at higher risk of developing hypertension or those who are already diagnosed with hypertension or those who are concerned about developing hypertension should adopt Healthy lifestyle habits. Those who are already diagnosed with hypertension should in addition to adopting healthy lifestyle habits adhere strictly to the prescriptions from their doctor.

i. Preventing High Blood Pressure Onset

Adopting healthy lifestyle habits can help prevent high blood pressure from developing. Since hypertension is a symptomless disease, people should make it a point of duty to check their blood pressure regularly. Children should have their blood pressure checked starting at 3 years of age. If prehypertension is detected, it should be taken seriously to avoid progressing to high blood pressure.

ii. Preventing Worsening High Blood Pressure or Complications

If anybody has been diagnosed with high blood pressure, it is important to obtain regular medical care and to follow the prescribed treatment plan, which will include healthy lifestyle habit recommendations and possibly medicines. Healthy lifestyle habits will not only prevent the development of high blood pressure but can also reverse prehypertension and help control existing high blood pressure to prevent complications and long-term problems associated with this condition, such as coronary heart disease, stroke, or kidney disease

2. **Treatment Plan:** Treatment plan depends on whether the individual is diagnosed with primary (essential) hypertension or secondary hypertension. If someone is diagnosed with secondary hypertension, treating the cause of the hypertension effectively could reverse the hypertension. In that case the person will only adopt healthy lifestyle habits without using any medications. If the individual is diagnosed with primary hypertension the treatment plan will include healthy lifestyle habits and medications.

Resistant hypertension is defined as hypertension that remains above goal blood pressure in spite of using, at once, three antihypertensive medications belonging to different drug classes and adopting a healthy lifestyle habit. Low adherence to treatment is an important cause of resistant hypertension. Resistant hypertension may also represent the result of chronic high activity of the autonomic nervous system; this concept is known as **"neurogenic hypertension"**.

This can happen when the medications that they are taking do not work well for them or another medical condition is leading to uncontrolled blood pressure. Treatment of resistant high blood pressure involves an intensive treatment plan that can include a different set of blood pressure medications or other special treatments.

Maintaining a controlled blood pressure is very important because it will not only prevent or delay complications of high blood pressure but can also lower the risk for other related problems.

Healthy Lifestyle Habits

What are these Healthy lifestyle habits? These habits include:

- **Healthy eating**

- **Being physically active**

- **Maintaining a healthy weight**

- **Limiting alcohol intake**

- **Managing and coping with stress**

Changes are difficult to make and adhere to. So to help make lifelong lifestyle changes, one has to try making one healthy lifestyle change at a time. When one is comfortable with that lifestyle change, another change will be added. Maximum benefit will be achieved by adopting many healthy lifestyle habits (at least five).

1. Healthy Eating

It is recommended that people should limit the amount of sodium chloride and increase the amount of potassium, calcium and magnesium that they consume. It is also recommended that people should eat food that are considered as being healthy for the heart.

Limiting Sodium and Salt

Salt intake should be between 2.**3 grams to 6 grams per day**. Very low salt intake or very high salt intake is not good for any individual whether hypertensive or not. It is recommended that people should avoid adding salt or seasonings on the table as these will lead to water retention and consequently an increase in blood volume, which is a factor in causing high blood pressure.

A "Dietary Approaches to Stop Hypertension (DASH)" eating plan is recommended for everybody whether hypertensive or not because it is good for the heart. The DASH eating plan focuses on **fruits, vegetables, whole grains, and other foods that are heart healthy and low in fat, cholesterol, and salt**.

Description of the DASH Eating Plan

DASH is a flexible and balanced eating plan that helps create a heart-healthy eating style for life.

The DASH eating plan requires no special foods and instead provides daily and weekly nutritional goals. This plan recommends:

- Eating vegetables, fruits, and whole grains

- Including fat-free or low-fat dairy products, fish, poultry, beans, nuts, and vegetable oils

- Limiting foods that are high in saturated fat, such as fatty meats, full-fat dairy products, and tropical oils such as coconut, palm kernel, and palm oils

- Limiting sugar-sweetened beverages and sweets.

Based on these recommendations, the following table shows examples of daily and weekly servings that meet DASH eating plan targets for a 2,000-calorie-a-day diet.

Daily and Weekly DASH Eating Plan Goals for a
2,000-Calorie-a-Day Diet

Food Group	Daily Servings
Grains	6–8
Meats, poultry, and fish	6 or less
Vegetables	4–5
Fruit	4–5
Low-fat or fat-free dairy products	2–3
Fats and oils	2–3
Sodium	2,300 mg*
	Weekly Servings
Nuts, seeds, dry beans, and	4–5

peas	
Sweets	5 or less

*1,500 milligrams (mg) sodium lowers blood pressure even further than 2,300 mg sodium daily.

When following the DASH eating plan, it is important to choose foods that are:

- Low in saturated and *trans* fats

- Rich in potassium, calcium, magnesium, fibre, and protein

- Lower in sodium

Potassium: Potassium is an essential nutrient used to maintain fluid and electrolyte balance in the body. A deficiency in potassium causes fatigue, irritability, and hypertension (high blood pressure). Overdose of potassium from natural sources is nearly impossible. However, it is possible to consume too much potassium via potassium salts. Overdose of potassium can lead to nausea, vomiting, and even cardiac arrest. Potassium from fruits, like the ones listed below, is considered safe and healthy. The current daily value for potassium is 3.5 grams.

Fruits rich in Potassium

Avocadoes, Guavas, Bananas, Passion fruit, Kiwi fruit, Persimmons, Cantaloupe melon, Apricots, Pomegranate, Figs, Honeydew melon, Cherries, Pummelos, Nectarines, Grapes, Peaches, Kumquats, Papaya (paw paw), Oranges, Clementines (or Tangerines), Litchis, Mangoes, Blackberries, Plums, Strawberries, Raspberries, Grapefruit, Lemons, Apples (Granny Smith), Pears, Watermelon, Pineapples, and Limes.

Vegetables high in Potassium:

Beet Greens (cooked), Yam, Garden Cress, Lima Beans (cooked), Spinach, Swiss chard (cooked), Potatoes (baked), Bamboo Shoots, Kale, Sweet Potato (cooked), Mushrooms (Brown), Jerusalem Artichokes, Fennel, Brussels Sprouts, Parsnip,

Pak Choi (Chinese Cabbage) cooked, Globe Artichokes, Arugula (Rocket), Squash (Winter), Broccoli Raab (Rapini) cooked, Pumpkin, Watercress, (Beets Beetroot), Snap Beans (Yellow) cooked, Carrots, Broccoli, Endive, Rutabagas (Swede), Celeriac, Cauliflower, Okra, Sweet Corn (Frozen), Celery (cooked).

Foods high in Potassium:

White Beans, Dark Leafy Greens (Spinach), Baked Potatoes (with skin), Dried Apricots, Baked Acorn Squash, Yogurt (Plain, Skim/Non-fat), Fish (salmon), Avocados, Mushroom (White) and Bananas.

Foods high in Calcium:

Almonds, Cabbage, Chinese cabbage (cooked), Cheese (firm, such as cheddar, mozzarella, provolone), Cheese (hard, such as parmesan, or pecorino), Collard Greens (cooked), Cottage cheese (2% milk fat), Figs (dried), Kale (cooked), Milk (whole), Mustard Greens (cooked), Salmon (canned with bones), Sardines (canned with bones), Sesame Seeds, Sesame Seed Butter (tahini), Spinach (cooked), Spices (cinnamon, cumin, basil, oregano, parsley, black pepper), Swiss Chard (cooked), and Yogurt (Plain, full fat)

Foods high in Magnesium:

Almonds, Artichoke, Brazil Nuts, Cashews, Dark chocolate, Fish (mackerel, halibut, cod), Flax Seeds, Molasses, Papaya, Potato (with skin), Pumpkin Seeds, Sesame Seeds, Spinach (cooked), Sunflower Seeds, Swiss Chard, and Tuna

Food good for the heart: (Heart-healthy eating)

- Whole grains

- Fruits, such as apples, bananas, oranges, pears, and prunes

- Vegetables, such as broccoli, cabbage, and carrots

- Legumes, such as kidney beans, lentils, chick peas, black-eyed peas, and lima beans

- Fat-free or low-fat dairy products, such as skim milk

- Fish high in omega-3 fatty acids, such as salmon, tuna, and trout, about twice a week

Avoid eating:

- A lot of red meat

- Palm and coconut oils;

- Sugary foods and beverages

2. Being Physically Active:

Routine physical activity can lower high blood pressure and reduce the risk for other health problems. It is important to consult a doctor before embarking on a new exercise plan. This consultation will help the person in making the right choice of exercise plan. For example, it will not be advisable for a person with a weak heart to start with vigorous aerobic exercises.

Everyone should try to participate in moderate-intensity aerobic exercise at least 2 hours and 30 minutes per week, or vigorous-intensity aerobic exercise for 1 hour and 15 minutes per week. Aerobic exercise, such as brisk walking, makes the heart beat harder and pump more blood and oxygen to the tissues and organs of the body. The more active a person is, the more he will benefit. Adults should participate in aerobic exercise for at least 10 minutes at a time, spread throughout the week.

3. Maintaining a Healthy Weight

Maintaining a healthy weight can help to control high blood pressure and reduce the risk for other health problems. Obese people should try to reduce weight. A small weight loss of just 3 to 5 percent can lower the risk for health problems. Greater amounts of weight loss can improve blood pressure readings, lower LDL cholesterol (bad cholesterol), and increase HDL cholesterol (good cholesterol).

A useful measure of overweight and obesity is body mass index (BMI). BMI measures the weight of an individual in relation to the height. BMI can be calculated using a BMI calculator found online. The interpretation of BMI is given below:

A Body mass index (BMI) that is

- Below 18.5 shows that the person is underweight.

- Between 18.5 and 24.9 is in the healthy range.

- Between 25 and 29.9 is considered overweight.

- Of 30 or more is considered obese.

Everybody should aim for a BMI of below 25.

Waist Circumference

Measuring waist circumference helps screen for possible health risks that come with overweight and obesity. Fat that is deposited around the waist rather than at the hips, signifies a higher risk for heart disease and type 2 diabetes. This risk goes up with a waist size that is greater than 35 inches (87.5 cm) for women or greater than 40 inches (100 cm) for men. To correctly measure the waist, the tape measure should be placed around the middle just above the hip bones (a little below the navel) when the person is standing up. Measurement should be done just after breathing out.

People who are overweight but do not have a high waist measurement, and have fewer than two risk factors may need to prevent further weight gain rather than lose weight.

Obesity is not only a risk factor for hypertension, it is also a risk factor for many other disease conditions like diabetes mellitus, heart attack, heart failure, sudden death and bone diseases.

4. Limiting Alcohol Intake:

It is important that alcohol intake should be reduced. Too much alcohol raises the blood pressure and triglyceride levels, (a type of fat found in the blood). Alcohol also adds extra calories, which may cause weight gain.

Men should have no more than two drinks containing alcohol a day. Women should have no more than one drink containing alcohol a day.

One drink is equal to:

- 355 ml of beer

- 150 ml of wine

- 45 ml of liquor

5. Managing and Coping With Stress

Stressful conditions are part of our everyday life, but some people manage stress better than others. Learning how to manage stress, relax, and cope with problems can improve one's emotional and physical health and can lower high blood pressure. Stress management techniques include:

- Being physically active

- Listening to music or focusing on something calm or peaceful

- Performing yoga or tai chi

- Meditating

Medications: (Medicines)

Medical management should be left for the healthcare team (doctors, nurses, pharmacists and other trained health personnel). Those who are diagnosed with hypertension should try to follow their doctor's prescriptions for maximum benefits.

The medicines for treating high blood pressure are grouped depending on their mode and site of action. It is the doctor who knows the best combination that will achieve the desired result with minimal adverse effects. The groups of medicines are:

- **Diuretics:** This group of medicines eliminates water and excess sodium from the body thereby reducing the blood volume and consequently the blood pressure.

- **Beta Blockers:** Medicines in this group help to reduce the heart rate and lessens the force of heart beat. As a result, the heart pumps less blood through the blood vessels, thereby helping to lower the blood pressure.

- **Angiotensin-Converting Enzyme (ACE) Inhibitors**: Angiotensin-II is a hormone that narrows blood vessels, and increases blood pressure. ACE converts Angiotensin I to Angiotensin II. ACE inhibitors block this conversion of Angiotensin-I to Angiotensin-II and consequently lower the blood pressure.

- **Angiotensin II Receptor Blockers (ARBs):** This group blocks angiotensin II hormone from binding with receptors in the blood vessels. When angiotensin II is blocked, the blood vessels do not constrict or narrow, which can lower the blood pressure.

- **Calcium Channel Blockers:** Medicines in this group prevent calcium from entering the heart muscles and blood vessels. This allows blood vessels to relax, and so lowers the blood pressure.

- **Alpha Blockers:** Reduce nerve impulses that tighten (constrict) blood vessels. This allows blood to flow more freely, causing blood pressure to go down.

- **Alpha-Beta Blockers:** Reduce nerve impulses the same way alpha blockers do. However, like beta blockers, they also slow the heartbeat. As a result, blood pressure goes down.

- **Central Acting Agents:** Act in the brain to decrease nerve signals that narrow blood vessels, thereby lowering the blood pressure.

- **Vasodilators:** These relax the muscles in blood vessel walls. Relaxing the blood vessel muscles reduces the peripheral resistance and consequently lowers the blood pressure.

Living with high blood pressure

For anybody who has high blood pressure, the best thing to do is to talk with their health care provider and take steps to control their blood pressure by making healthy lifestyle changes and taking medications, if any have been prescribed for them.

For a healthy future, it is important for the people who have high blood pressure to follow their treatment plan closely and work with their health care team.

It is important to adopt and follow **Healthy Lifestyle Changes** like:

- Follow a healthy diet.

- Be physically active.

- Maintain a healthy weight.

- Limit alcohol intake.

- Stop smoking for those who are smoking.

- Get plenty of sleep.

- Drink more water.

All these measures will go a long way in controlling high blood pressure.

Medicines

It is important to take all blood pressure medicines as prescribed by the health care provider. Know the names and doses of the medicines and how to take them. Refer all questions about your medicines to the health care provider or pharmacist. Make sure to refill the medicines before they run out; don't spend a day without medications. Take the medicines exactly as prescribed by the health care provider.

Ongoing Care

It is very important to keep track of the blood pressure. Those who can afford, could buy the machine to check their blood pressure at home. They should keep a logbook for the blood pressure and go for check-ups with the logbook. It is important to do regular eye checks with a qualified personnel. To check blood sugar levels for diabetes regularly. It is also important to discuss all health concerns with the healthcare provider during check-ups to obtain accurate information. Wrong information from family and friends could be detrimental. Any changes in the medications should only be done by the healthcare provider.

Pregnancy Planning

High blood pressure can cause problems for mother and baby. High blood pressure can harm the mother's kidneys and other organs and can cause early (premature) birth and low birth weight. So any woman who has high blood pressure and is planning to have a baby is advised to discuss with her healthcare team so that appropriate steps should be taken to control the blood pressure before and during the pregnancy.

Some women develop high blood pressure during pregnancy (pregnancy-induced hypertension). When this happens, the health care provider will closely monitor the woman and her baby and provide special care to lower the chance of complications. With such care, most women and babies have good outcomes.

Chapter Five

Useful health tips

- Cleanliness is key to good health.

- Wash hands always before eating anything.

- Wash hands after using the bathrooms.

- Wash hands after touching anything like the door handles and railings.

- Wash hands when coming from the outside.

- Wash hands after touching garbage or dirty laundry.

- Wash hands before preparing and after eating food.

- Wash hands after touching animals or pets.

- Wash hands after blowing nose or sneezing.

- Wash hands after changing a baby's diapers or touching any soiled item.

- When washing hands, pay particular attention to the fingernails and between the fingers.

- Dry hands with disposable paper towel or tissue paper; don't use towel used by another person or other persons.

- In the absence of something to dry the hands, hold them out in the air to dry.

- Don't touch anything with wet hands; you will contaminate whatever it is.

- Wash fruits well before eating.

- Wash fruits and vegetables well before cooking.

- Cooking destroys the vitamin C in the fruits, so eat fruits raw for more vitamin C.

- Always use clean water for washing.

- Brush teeth at least twice a day.

- Take bath at least once every day.

- Don't wear dirty clothes; they smell and can cause skin disease and rash.

- Open windows at home to allow in fresh air.

- Drink a cup of water at room temperature first thing in the morning.

- Eat more vegetables than carbohydrates in every meal.

- Avoid sugary beverages.

- Hot and spicy food is not good for people who have peptic ulcer.

- Alcohol is not good for peptic ulcer sufferers.

- Cigarette smoking is not good for pregnant women; it could damage their babies.

- Do physical exercise every day. (At least walk for thirty minutes every day).

- Avoid too much alcohol; it can damage your heart, liver or kidney.

- Avoid cigarette smoking, but if you must smoke, don't smoke in a closed place.

- Eat your food steamed, broiled, grilled or cooked; avoid frying all the time.

- Avoid the use of solid fats.

- Trim fingernails and toenails regularly

- Visit the clinic for routine check-up at least every two months.

- Visit the dentist at least twice a year.

- Visit the eye doctor (ophthalmologist) at least once a year for routine check.

- Any woman above the age of twenty five years must do Pap smear every five years, but more frequently if she is HIV positive. Pap smear is a test to detect cancer of the cervix early. Cancer of the cervix is curable if detected early.

- Every woman must examine her breast for lumps regularly. Any lump must be reported to the doctor immediately. Breast cancer is curable if detected early but it is a death sentence if detected late.

- Have at least six hours of sleep every night.

- Smile always.

- Getting enough rest both physically and mentally every day is good for health.

- Release negative thoughts.

- Don't lift heavy objects from the side; always lift from in front. Lifting from the side could damage your waist.

- Tree nuts (like cashew, almond and hazel) and legume nuts like peanuts are good for health.

- Banana, beans, dark leafy green, avocados, fish, yoghurt, potatoes etc. are rich in potassium and are good for health especially for people who have hypertension.

- People, who want to lose weight should stick to three meals a day (should not eat between meals), reduce the quantity of food, eat more portions of fruits and vegetables than starchy food. Eat less fatty, salty and sugary meals. Exercise daily.

- Oils that are liquid at room temperature like vegetable oil and olive oil are better than oils that are solid at room temperature like fats and margarine.

- Ladies should not use toilet paper or piece of cloth as sanitary pad; it breeds infection.

- Wash pair of socks after every use.

References:

1. *White WB (May 2009). "Defining the problem of treating the patient with hypertension and arthritis pain". The American Journal of Medicine. **122** (5 Suppl): S3–9.doi:10.1016/j.amjmed.2009.03.002. PMID 19393824. Retrieved 2009-06-22.*

2. *Organization. Global Health Observatory (GHO) data.*

3. *Kearney PM, Whelton M, Reynolds K, Muntner P, Whelton PK, He J; Whelton; Reynolds; Muntner; Whelton; He (2005). "Global burden of hypertension: analysis of worldwide data".Lancet. 365 (9455): 217–23. doi:10.1016/S0140-6736(05)17741-1. PMID 15652604.*

4. *Kearney PM, Whelton M, Reynolds K, Whelton PK, He J; Whelton; Reynolds; Whelton; He (January 2004). "Worldwide*

prevalence of hypertension: a systematic review". J. Hypertens. 22 (1): 11–9. doi:10.1097/00004872-200401000-00003. PMID 15106785.

5. *Burt VL, Whelton P, Roccella EJ, et al. (March 1995). "Prevalence of hypertension in the US adult population. Results from the Third National Health and Nutrition Examination Survey, 1988–1991". Hypertension. 25 (3): 305–13. doi:10.1161/01.HYP.25.3.305.PMID 7875754. Retrieved 5 June 2009.*

6. *Burt VL, Cutler JA, Higgins M, et al. (July 1995). "Trends in the prevalence, awareness, treatment, and control of hypertension in the adult US population. Data from the health examination surveys, 1960 to 1991". Hypertension. 26 (1): 60–9.doi:10.1161/01.HYP.26.1.60. PMID 7607734. Retrieved 5 June 2009.*

7. *Ostchega Y, Dillon CF, Hughes JP, Carroll M, Yoon S; Dillon; Hughes; Carroll; Yoon (July*

2007). "Trends in hypertension prevalence, awareness, treatment, and control in older U.S. adults: data from the National Health and Nutrition Examination Survey 1988 to 2004".Journal of the American Geriatrics Society. 55 (7): 1056–65. doi:10.1111/j.1532-5415.2007.01215.x. PMID 17608879.

8. Lloyd-Jones D, Adams RJ, Brown TM, et al. (February 2010). "Heart disease and stroke statistics--2010 update: a report from the American Heart Association". Circulation.121 (7): e46–e215. doi:10.1161/CIRCULATIONAHA.109.1926 67. PMID 20019324.

9. "Culture-Specific of Health Risk Health Status: Morbidity and Mortality". Stanford. Retrieved 12 April 2016.

10. Agabiti-Rosei E (September 2008). "From macro- to microcirculation: benefits in hypertension and diabetes". Journal of Hypertension Supplement. 26 (3): S15–

9.*doi*:*10.1097/01.hjh.0000334602.71005.52*.
PMID *19363848*

11. *Rodriguez-Cruz, Edwin; Ettinger, Leigh M (April 6, 2010). "Hypertension".eMedicine Pediatrics: Cardiac Disease and Critical Care Medicine. Medscape. Retrieved16 June 2009.*

12. *Falkner B (May 2009). "Hypertension in children and adolesents: epidemiology and natural history". Pediatr. Nephrol. 25 (7): 1219–24. doi:10.1007/s00467-009-1200-3.PMC 2874036 . PMID 19421783.*

13. *Luma GB, Spiotta RT; Spiotta (May 2006). "Hypertension in children and adolescents".Am Fam Physician. 73 (9): 1558–68. PMID 16719248.*

14. *Schrader J (April 2009). "[Stroke and hypertension]". Der Internist (in German). 50 (4): 423–32. doi:10.1007/s00108-008-2291-9. PMID 19308341.*

15. *Zeng C, Villar VA, Yu P, Zhou L, Jose PA (April 2009). "Reactive oxygen species and dopamine receptor function in essential*

hypertension". Clinical and Experimental Hypertension. **31** *(2): 156–78. doi:10.1080/10641960802621283. PMID 19330604. Retrieved 2009-06-20.*

16. *Varon J (October 2007). "Diagnosis and management of labile blood pressure during acute cerebrovascular accidents and other hypertensive crises". The American Journal of Emergency Medicine.* **25** *(8): 949–59. doi:10.1016/j.ajem.2007.02.032.PMID 17 920983. Retrieved 2009-06-20.*

17. *Sare GM, Geeganage C, Bath PM (2009). "High blood pressure in acute ischaemic stroke--broadening therapeutic horizons". Cerebrovascular Diseases.* **27 Suppl** *1: 156–61. doi:10.1159/000200454. PMID 19342846. Retrieved 2009-06-20.*

18. *Palm F, Urbanek C, Grau A (April 2009). "Infection, its treatment and the risk for stroke". Current Vascular Pharmacology.* **7** *(2): 146–*

52.doi:10.2174/15701610978745707. PMID 19355997. Retrieved 2009-06-20.

19. Tanahashi N (April 2009). "[Roles of angiotensin II receptor blockers in stroke prevention]". Nippon Rinsho (in Japanese). 67 (4): 742–9. PMID 19348237.

20. Walsh JB (October 1982). "Hypertensive retinopathy. Description, classification, and prognosis". Ophthalmology. 89 (10): 1127–31. doi:10.1016/s0161-6420(82)34664-3.PMID 7155523.

21. Liebreich R. Ophthalmoskopischer Befund bei Morbus Brightii. Albrecht von Graefes Arch Ophthalmol 1859; 5: 265–268.

22. Tso MO, Jampol LM (October 1982). "Pathophysiology of hypertensive retinopathy".Ophthalmology. 89 (10): 1132–45. doi:10.1016/s0161-6420(82)34663-1.PMID 7155524.

23. Wong TY, Mitchell P (November 2004). "Hypertensive retinopathy". The New England Journal of Medicine. 351 (22): 2310–

7. *doi:10.1056/NEJMra032865*. *PMID 15564 546*. *Retrieved 2009-06-24.*

24. *Pache M, Kube T, Wolf S, Kutschbach P (June 2002). "Do angiographic data support a detailed classification of hypertensive fundus changes?". Journal of Human Hypertension.**16** (6): 405– 10. doi:10.1038/sj.jhh.1001402. PMID 12037 695.*

25. *Krzesinski JM, Cohen EP (2007). "Hypertension and the kidney". Acta Clinica Belgica. **62(1)**: 5–14. PMID 17451140.*

26. *Monhart V (May 2008). "[Diabetes mellitus, hypertension and kidney]". Vnitřní Lékařství(in Czech). **54** (5): 499–504, 507. PMID 18630636.*

27. *Hohenstein K, Watschinger B (2008). "[Hypertension and the kidney]". Wiener Medizinische Wochenschrift (in German). **158** (13–14): 359– 64. doi:10.1007/s10354-008-0558-3. PMID 18677585.*

28. *Khosla N, Kalaitzidis R, Bakris GL (May 2009). "The kidney, hypertension, and remaining challenges". The Medical Clinics of North America.* **93** *(3): 697–715, Table of Contents.doi:10.1016/j.mcna.2009.02.001. PMID 19427500. Retrieved 2009-06-23.*

29. *Ponnuchamy B, Khalil RA (April 2009). "Cellular mediators of renal vascular dysfunction in hypertension". American Journal of Physiology.* **296** *(4): R1001–18.doi:10.1152/ajpregu.90960.2008. PMC 2698613. PMID 19225145. Retrieved2009-06-23.*

30. *Niang A (2008). "[Arterial hypertension and the kidney]". Dakar Médical (in French).* **53***(1): 1–6. PMID 19102111.*

31. *Palmer BF (October 2008). "Hypertension management in patients with chronic kidney disease". Current Hypertension Reports.* **10** *(5): 367–73. doi:10.1007/s11906-008-0069-z. PMID 18775113.*

32. Gibson, Paul (July 30, 2009). _"Hypertension and Pregnancy"_. eMedicine Obstetrics and Gynecology. Medscape. Retrieved 16 June 2009.

33. Marín R, Gorostidi M, Fernández-Vega F, Alvarez-Navascués R (December 2005). "Systemic and glomerular hypertension and progression of chronic renal disease: the dilemma of nephrosclerosis". _Kidney International Supplement_. **68** (99): S52–6._doi_:_10.1111/j.1523-1755.2005.09910.x_. _PMID_ _16336577_.

34. Schmitz A (September 1997). "Microalbuminuria, blood pressure, metabolic control, and renal involvement: longitudinal studies in white non-insulin-dependent diabetic patients"._American Journal of Hypertension_. **10** (9 Pt 2): 189S–197S. _doi_:_10.1016/S0895-7061(97)00152-0_. _PMID_ _9324121_.

35. Hennersdorf MG, Strauer BE (March 2006). "[Hypertension and heart]"._Medizinische_

Klinik (in German). 101 Suppl 1: 27–30. PMID 16802514.

36. *Hennersdorf MG, Strauer BE (March 2007). "[The heart in hypertension]". Der Internist (in German). 48 (3): 236–45. doi:10.1007/s00108-006-1762-0.PMID 17260148.*

37. *Motz W (October 2004). "[Right ventricle in arterial hypertension]". Der Internist (in German). 45 (10): 1108–16. doi:10.1007/s00108-004-1273-9. PMID 15351931.*

38. *Wachtell K, Devereux RB, Lyle PA, Okin PM, Gerdts E (December 2008). "The left atrium, atrial fibrillation, and the risk of stroke in hypertensive patients with left ventricular hypertrophy". Therapeutic Advances in Cardiovascular Disease. 2 (6): 507–13.doi:10.1177/1753944708093846. PMID 19124445. Retrieved 2009-06-22.*

39. *Petrović D, Stojimirović B (2008). "[Left ventricular hypertrophy in patients treated with regular hemodialyses]". Medicinski Pregled (in*

Serbian). **61** *(7–8): 369–*
74.doi:10.2298/MPNS0808369P. PMID 1909
7374.

40. *Cuspidi C, Sala C, Zanchetti A (December*
    2007). "Management of hypertension in
    patients with left ventricular
    hypertrophy". Current Hypertension
    Reports. **9** *(6): 498–505.doi:10.1007/s11906-*
    007-0091-6. PMID 18367014.

41. *Simko F (September 2007). "Statins: a*
    perspective for left ventricular hypertrophy
    treatment". European Journal of Clinical
    Investigation. **37** *(9): 681–*
    91.doi:10.1111/j.1365-
    2362.2007.01837.x. PMID 17696957.
    Retrieved 2009-06-22.

42. *Wachtell K, Devereux RB, Lyle AP (August*
    2007). "The effect of angiotensin receptor
    blockers for preventing atrial
    fibrillation". Current Hypertension
    Reports. **9** *(4): 278–83.doi:10.1007/s11906-*
    007-0051-1. PMID 17686377.

43. *Herpin D (March 1999). "[Impact of arterial hypertension on the heart]". La Revue du praticien (in French).* **49** *(5): 491– 4. PMID 10358398.*

44. *Diabetes and Hypertension Medical Journal of Australia. 2010-02-09*

45. *Diabetes associated to Hypertension About health portal. 2010-02-09*

46. *Medical journal of Australia. "Hypertension and Diabetes overview" 2010-02-09.*

47. *http://www.nhlbi.nih.gov/health/health-topics/topics/hbp/preventionSep 10, 2015 ... **Prevention of High Blood Pressure**. Healthy lifestyle habits, proper use of medicines, and regular medical care can prevent high blood pressure ...*

48. *http://www.heart.org/HEARTORG/Conditions/HighBloodPressure/PreventionTreatmentofHighBloodPressure/Prevention-Treatment-of-High-Blood-Pressure_UCM_002054_Article.jspJun 29, 2016 ... The American Heart Association*

*explains the **prevention of high blood pressure**, also called hypertension, and the treatment of high blood ..*

BOUT THE AUTHOR

Dr Bennett Onyebuchukwu Obi is a Nigerian born at Oraifite in Anambra state. He attended Oraifite Grammar School for his secondary education. He is an alumnus of the University of Nigeria Nsukka in Nigeria and the University of Stellenbosch in South Africa. He specialized in the HIV/AIDS management. He is married with three children. He has worked in many different parts of Nigeria (Anambra state, Cross river state, Kwara state and Federal Capital Territory Abuja). He has also worked in the Comoros islands, Kenya and Lesotho. He has so many other titles to his credit: The Villager, Before the Dawn, Tales of Our Time, The Conscript, Gem in a Rubbish Heap, Sacrifice (I made for my child), Essential Health Basics for Developing Countries, Preventable Tsunami, Stop and Ponder (because nothing happens by chance), Cry of the Innocent, The Alma Mater, Isabella My Sweet Angel, Igbo Cultural Heritage; A vanishing Identity, My Goodwill; My Nemesis, the Amoral Country and Double Swap.